NURSING ESSENTIALS
Drugs

CATRIN PAGE

Doctor
General Medicine
United Kingdom

Translated by
Bronwen Davies
Watership Translations

ELSEVIER

ELSEVIER

Edinburgh London New York Oxford Philadelphia St Louis Sydney 2020

© 2020, Elsevier Limited. All rights reserved.

First published in Germany under the title:

Taschenwissen Pflege Arzneimittellehre
ISBN Print 978-3-437-25332-4
ISBN e-Book 978-3-437-18834-3

Elsevier GmbH, Urban & Fischer Verlag
Hackerbrücke 6, 80335 München
Germany

This translation of *Taschenwissen Pflege Arzneimittellehre*, by Dr. Catrin Page was undertaken by Elsevier Ltd and is published by arrangement with Elsevier Inc.

Nursing Essentials: Drugs, Translated and Adapted Edition.

ISBN: 978-0-7020-7763-0

Printed in China

Last digit is the print number: 9 8 7 6 5 4 3 2 1

Content Strategist: Poppy Garraway Smith, Serena Castelnovo
Content Development Specialist: Carole McMurray
Content Coordinator: Kirsty Guest
Project Manager: Beula Christopher
Design: Amy Buxton
Marketing Manager: Kristen Oyirifi

Contents

Abbreviations

ADR	Adverse drug reaction(s), side effect(s)		INR	International Normalized Ratio
ASA	Acetylsalicylic acid, aspirin		MAO inhibitors	Monoamine oxidase inhibitors
BG	Blood glucose, blood sugar		Min.	Minute(s)
BP	Blood pressure (RR: Riva-Rocci)		NSAID	Non-steroidal anti-inflammatory drug
ca.	circa, approximately		OP	Operation
CD	Controlled Drug		Pat.	Patient
CHD (alt: CAD)	Coronary heart disease, coronary artery disease		poss.	Possibly, maybe
			St.p.	Status post
chron.	Chronic		Supp.	Suppository
CK	Creatine kinase		Tab	Tablet(s)
CNS	Central nervous system		TIA	Transient ischaemic attack
COPD	Chronic obstructive pulmonary disease		&	and
Diab.	Diabetes		/d	Per day, daily
e.g.	For example		↑	Increased, elevated
HL	Half-life		→	Consequently
Hr	Hour		↓	Decreased
i.m.	Intramuscular(ly)			
i.v.	Intravenous(ly)			
IMI	Injection-meal interval			

Antiarrhythmic drugs Antiarrhythmic drugs = medicines used in the treatment of cardiac arrhythmias.

Tab. 1 Antiarrhythmic drugs

Active ingredient/ trade name	Indications	Contraindications	Side effects	Comments
Atropine Atropine sulfate	• Acute bradyarrhythmias (short-term therapy) • Antidote for poisoning with parasympathomimetic drugs • Gastrointestinal and urogenital spasms • Inhibition of secretion in the stomach and pancreas	• Narrow-angle glaucoma • Tachycardia • Gastrointestinal obstruction • Coronary stenosis • Prostatic enlargement • Bladder dysfunction • Acute pulmonary oedema • Preeclampsia • Last trimester of pregnancy	• Gastrointestinal disorders • Visual disturbances • Hyperthermia • Urinary retention • Dry mouth • Tachycardia • Restlessness, hallucinations	• Use only under constant ECG and vital signs monitoring • Atropine is an antimuscarinic agent causing unwanted side effects listed
Lidocaine	• Approved as a local and regional nerve block	• Severe cardiac conduction disturbances • Acute decompensated heart failure • Heart attack in the last 3 months • Cardiogenic or hypovolaemic shock	• Dizziness • Paraesthesia • Drowsiness • BP ↓ • Arrhythmia	Only for short-term treatment

BP, blood pressure; *ECG*, electrocardiogram

Cardiac glycosides Cardiac glycosides = naturally occurring medicine that is bound to a steroid derivative. They have a positive inotropic effect on the heart.

Tab. 2 Cardiac glycosides

Active ingredient/ trade names	Indications	Contraindications	Side effects	Comments
Digoxin Lanicor	• Chronic heart failure • Atrial fibrillation/flutter with rapid ventricular response • Paroxysmal atrial fibrillation/flutter • Treatment and prevention of paroxysmal supraventricular tachycardia	• Sick sinus syndrome • AV block grades II and III • Ventricular tachycardia and fibrillation • Wolf-Parkinson-White (WPW) syndrome • Hypercalcaemia • Hypokalaemia • Hypertrophic obstructive cardiomyopathy	• Nausea, vomiting, diarrhoea • Bradycardia, arrhythmias • Confusion, agitation, depression, headache, fatigue, insomnia • Signs of overdose: changes in colour vision, visual changes	• Potency can be affected by many medications and varying electrolyte concentrations • Narrow therapeutic index, therefore need to monitor serum levels and if necessary, adjust digoxin dose

Calcium channel blockers Calcium channel blockers = medicines that inhibit the transport of Ca^{2+} into cells; they act on vascular smooth muscle cells → vasodilation → BP ↓, relaxation of the heart.

Tab. 3 Calcium channel blockers

Active ingredient/ trade names	Indications	Contraindications	Side effects	Comments
Amiodarone	Symptomatic supraventricular and ventricular tachyarrhythmias (including atrial fibrillation)	• Hypersensitivity to amiodarone • Iodine allergy • Sinus bradycardia • Cardiac conduction delays • Thyroid disease • Preexisting QT prolongation • Hypokalaemia • Concomitant treatment with MAO inhibitors	• Thyroid disorders • Hyperpigmentation • Bradycardia • Acute hepatitis • Sleep disorders • Muscle weakness • Extrapyramidal tremor • Visual problems (corneal opacities) • Photosensitivity • Nerve damage • Pulmonary infiltrates and impaired pulmonary function	• Class I to IV antiarrhythmic agent (effect on: Na^+-, Ca^{2+}-, K^+ channels) • Avoid sunlight/tanning beds (even after discontinuing as long half-life) • Watch out for breathing problems (possible toxic effect on the lungs)

Active ingredient/ trade names	Indications	Contraindications	Side effects	Comments
Amlodipine	• Prophylaxis of angina • Essential hypertension	• Hypersensitivity to amlodipine • Cardiogenic shock • Severe aortic stenosis • Unstable angina pectoris • Acute heart attack • Severe hepatic impairment • Pregnancy: weight up risks versus benefits before prescribing • Breastfeeding	• Flushing • Feeling hot • Allergic reactions • Headache • Gastrointestinal complaints • Ankle swelling • Dizziness, drowsiness, weakness • Changes in visual perception	• Dihydropyridine type calcium channel blocker • Safe to take alongside β-blockers
Nifedipine	• Essential hypertension • Hypertensive emergency	• Hypersensitivity to nifedipine • Unstable angina pectoris • Cardiogenic shock • Acute heart attack • Pregnancy (avoid in first 20 weeks)/breastfeeding	• Gastrointestinal complaints • Fatigue, nervousness • Dizziness, tremor, neuropathy • Development or worsening of heart failure • Allergic reactions • Headache • Tinnitus	Dihydropyridine type calcium channel blocker

Active ingredient/ trade names	Indications	Contraindications	Side effects	Comments
Verapamil Isoptin	• Coronary heart disease (CAD) • Paroxysmal supraventricular tachycardia • Atrial fibrillation/flutter with rapid AV conduction • Hypertension	• Hypersensitivity to verapamil • Sick sinus syndrome • Cardiogenic shock • Acute heart attack with complications • Pronounced conduction disorders • Pregnancy • Overt heart failure	→ Nifedipine	• Phenylalkylamine type calcium blocker • To be taken whole with food • Do not take tablets lying down • Cannot take with β-blockers

β-blockers β-Blockers = medicines that have an affinity to β-receptors of the sympathetic nervous system.

Tab. 4 β-Blockers

Active ingredient/ trade names	Indications	Contraindications	Side effects	Comments
Carvedilol	• Essential hypertension • Chronic stable angina pectoris • Stable symptomatic, chronic heart failure	• Hypersensitivity • Recent heart attack • Bradycardia • Sick sinus syndrome • Atrioventricular (AV) block grade II and III • Sinoatrial block • Shock • Acidosis • Hypotension • Bronchial hyperresponsiveness • Severe peripheral circulatory disorders	• Arrhythmia • Vasoconstriction • Increased airway resistance • Dizziness, sweating, fatigue • Gastrointestinal complaints	• To be taken whole before meals • Treatment in small doses to start with then gradually increased • Close monitoring of pulse and, in the case of diabetics additional blood glucose monitoring, especially at the start of treatment • To be used cautiously in patients with asthma
Bisoprolol	• Hypertension • Coronary artery disease (CAD)	→ Carvedilol	→ Carvedilol	→ Carvedilol

Active ingredients/ trade names	Indications	Contraindications	Side effects	Comments
Metoprolol	• Chronic mild to moderate heart failure • Angina pectoris • Hypertension • Tachyarrhythmias • Migraine prophylaxis	• Bronchospasm • Bradycardia	• Headache • Bradycardia • Balance disorders • Palpitations • Sensation of coldness in extremities • Exertional dyspnoea • Gastrointestinal complaints	To be taken whole after meals
Sotalol	• Tachyarrhythmias (particularly paroxysmal atrial fibrillation)		• Fatigue, dizziness • Confusion • Anxiety • Headache • Chest pain • Taste disorders • Vision problems • Dry mouth • Muscle cramps	Tablets are taken whole before meals

Antihypertensives Antihypertensives = medicines used in the treatment of high blood pressure.

Tab. 5 Antihypertensives

Active ingredient/ trade names	Indications	Contraindications	Side effects	Comments
Enalapril/Ramipril	• Hypertension • Chronic heart failure in combination with diuretics and possibly cardiac glycosides and β-blockers • Prophylaxis following a heart attack • Diabetic nephropathy with macroproteinuria in patients with type I diabetes	• Hypersensitivity to the active ingredient or other ACE inhibitors • A history of angio-oedema • Renal artery stenosis • Pregnancy/breastfeeding • Lithium therapy	• Dry cough (reversible after discontinuing) • Gastrointestinal disorders • Hypotension • Dizziness, blurred vision • Headache • Rash, alopecia • Renal impairment • Tachyarrhythmia • Angina pectoris • Chest pain • Angio-oedema (rare, but life-threatening) • Taste disorders • Blood count problems	• If the patient has salt or volume depletion, has suffered a heart attack or severe hypertension, start with the smallest single dose • Enalapril and Ramipril are ACE inhibitors

Active ingredient/ trade names	Indications	Contraindications	Side effects	Comments
α-Methyldopa	• Pregnancy-induced hypertension • Essential hypertension, in combination with other antihypertensives (particularly diuretics)	• Hypersensitivity to methyldopa • Severe heart failure • Liver disease • Severe renal impairment • Phaeochromocytoma • A history of depression	• Sleepiness, drowsiness • Dizziness, fever • Dry mouth • Orthostatic hypotension • Oedema • Gastrointestinal disorders • Skin reactions • Erectile dysfunction • Gynaecomastia • Galactorrhoea	• Dark urine • α-methyldopa is an α-adrenergic receptor agonist

Active ingredient/ trade names	Indications	Contraindications	Side effects	Comments
Valsartan	• Essential hypertension • Treatment of heart failure following recent heart attack • Heart failure if ACE inhibitors or β-blockers are contraindicated	• Hypersensitivity to Valsartan • Severe hepatic failure, biliary cirrhosis and cholestasis • Severe renal failure • Pregnancy/breastfeeding	• Dizziness • Angio-oedema • Indigestion, digestive disorders • Muscle pain/cramps • Hyperkalaemia • Feeling of weakness/fatigue • Dyspnoea • Hypotension • Headache • Gastrointestinal complaints • Skin reactions • Urea in blood ↑, serum creatinine ↑ • Oedema • Angina pectoris • Palpitations • Insomnia • Cough • Constipation	• Absorption impaired by food by up to 40% • This is a type of antihypertensive that works as an angiotensin receptor blocker
Irbesartan	• Essential hypertension • Treatment of kidney disease in patients with hypertension and type II diabetes as part of antihypertensive treatment	• Hypersensitivity to irbesartan • Renal artery stenosis • Aortic or mitral (valve) stenosis • Obstructive hypertrophic cardiomyopathy • Pregnancy/breastfeeding		• This is a type of antihypertensive that works as an angiotensin receptor blocker

Active ingredients/ trade names	Indications	Contraindications	Side effects	Comments
• **Candesartan**	• Essential hypertension • Heart failure and impaired left ventricular systolic function in addition to ACE inhibitors or in the case of ACE inhibitor intolerance	• Hypersensitivity to candesartan • Severe liver damage and/or cholestasis • Renal artery stenosis • Aortic or mitral (valve) stenosis • Obstructive hypertrophic cardiomyopathy • Pregnancy/breastfeeding	→ Valsartan	This is a type of antihypertensive that works as an angiotensin receptor blocker
• **Olmesartan**	Essential hypertension	• Biliary obstruction • Renal artery stenosis • Impaired renal and hepatic function • Aortic or mitral (valve) stenosis • Obstructive hypertrophic cardiomyopathy • Concomitant use of lithium • Pregnancy/breastfeeding	→ Valsartan	This is a type of antihypertensive that works as an angiotensin receptor blocker

Active ingredient/ trade names	Indications	Contraindications	Side effects	Comments
Clonidine Catapresan	Hypertension unless caused by a phaeochromocytoma	• Hypersensitivity to clonidine • Cardiac de/repolarization and conduction disorders • Bradycardia • Pregnancy: risks versus benefit must be considered before prescribing • Breastfeeding	• Sedation • Dry mouth • Dry eyes • Drying out of nasal mucous membranes • Sleep disorders, nightmares • Perception disorders • Orthostatic hypotension • Oedema • Gastrointestinal disorders • Skin reactions • Erectile dysfunction	• Can also be administered subcutaneously and sublingually • Clonidine is an α-adrenoreceptor agonist

Anticoagulants Anticoagulants = medicines that reduce fibrin clot formation. Secondary haemostasis is disrupted.

! *Risk of bleeding in patients receiving anticoagulants! Always ensure that international normalised ratio (INR) and prothrombin time are regularly measured!*

Tab. 6 Anticoagulants

Active ingredient/ trade names	Indications	Contraindications	Side effects	Comments
Coumarins				
Warfarin	• Treatment and prophylaxis of thrombosis and embolism • Long-term anticoagulation • Used to reduce the risk of stroke in patients with atrial fibrillation	• Hypersensitivity to warfarin • Disorders associated with an increased bleeding tendency • Disorders where there is a suspected lesion in the vascular system • Recent surgery • Intramuscular (I.M) injections, lumbar punctures, regional anaesthesia with a spinal anaesthetic, angiograms • Pregnancy/breastfeeding	• (Gastrointestinal) bleeding • Nosebleeds, haematuria • Bleeding gums • Severe haematoma following trauma • Skin necrosis on breasts, hips, bottom, thigh • Jaundice • Gastrointestinal disorders • Hair loss	• Dosage depends on the current INR • Anticoagulant effect sets in after approx. 36–72 hours; if rapid anticoagulation is necessary, treatment with heparin must be initiated

Active substance/ trade names	Indications	Contraindications	Side effects	Comments
Direct oral anticoagulants				
Apixiban (Eliquis) Rivaroxaban Dabigatran	• Prophylaxis of venous thromboembolism following knee or hip replacement surgery • Prophylaxis of recurrent deep vein thrombosis or pulmonary embolism • Treatment of deep vein thrombosis or pulmonary embolism • Prophylaxis of stroke and embolism in nonvalvular atrial fibrillation	• Clinically significant bleeding • Gastrointestinal ulceration • High-risk bleeding cancers • Recent stroke • Recent brain or spinal surgery • Severe liver disease	• Bleeding (gastrointestinal or intracranial) • Rash • Bruising • Anaemia	

Active substance/ trade names	Indications	Contraindications	Side effects	Comments
Low molecular weight heparins (LMWHs)				
Dalteparin Fragmin **Tinzaparin** Enoxaparin clexane	• Prophylaxis of deep vein thrombosis in high-risk patients (e.g. postoperatively) • Treatment for deep vein thrombosis and pulmonary embolism • Prevention of reoccurring severe angina pectoris or an impending heart attack in patients with unstable angina pectoris and elevation myocardial infarction • Prophylaxis of vascular occlusions in hip operations and general surgical procedures in the abdominal region • Primary prophylaxis of venous thrombosis in patients with acute ischaemic stroke	The following contraindications apply to **all** LMWH: • Heparin-induced immune thrombocytopenia • Haemorrhagic diathesis • Acute haemorrhagic stroke or one going back less than 6 months or other intracranial bleeding • Active, clinically significant bleeding • Intracranial disorders • Gastrointestinal ulcers • Injuries or surgery on the central nervous system (CNS), eyes or ears • Uncontrollable severe hypertension • Severe hepatic and renal impairment • Disorders associated with an increased bleeding tendency • Disorders where there is a suspected lesion in the vascular system • Neonates, in particular immature preterm babies • Severe pancreatic disorders	• Dose-dependent overt or occult bleeding complications in various parts of the body • Subcutaneous haematoma, erythema, irritations at the injection site • Mild transient thrombocytopenia • Transaminases ↑ • Hypertension • Gastrointestinal complaints • Allergic reactions	• Can be given prophylactically or as treatment doses • Prefilled syringe with safety system: as soon as syringe is emptied, the needle draws back into inside the safety system

Antiplatelet drugs   Antiplatelet drugs = medicines that inhibit the aggregation of platelets in the arteries. Primary haemostasis is disrupted.

Tab. 7 Antiplatelet drugs

Active ingredient/ trade names	Indications	Contraindications	Side effects	Comments
Acetylsalicylic acid Aspirin	Antiplatelet therapy: • In the event of unstable angina pectoris • In the event of acute heart attack • For reinfarction prophylaxis • Following coronary artery stenting or other interventional procedures • For prophylaxis of transient ischaemic attacks (TIAs) and cerebral infarctions (stroke)	• Hypersensitivity to salicylates or other non-steroidal anti inflammatory drugs (NSAIDs) • Gastrointestinal ulcers • Asthma • Hepatic and renal failure • Severe heart failure • Caution with children (caution: Reye syndrome), in pregnancy/ breastfeeding and before surgery	• Gastrointestinal complaints, e.g. heartburn, nausea • Gastrointestinal bleeding • Allergies • Narrowing of the airways, particularly in the case of asthmatics	• Consider giving a proton pump inhibitor to protect the stomach from aspirin-induced gastritis
Clopidogrel	• Prevention of thrombo-embolism in patients with ischaemic stroke, heart attack or peripheral arterial disease and in acute coronary syndrome	• Hypersensitivity to clopidogrel • Severe renal and hepatic impairment • Acute pathologic bleeding	• Haematoma • Haematuria • Eye bleeding • Neutropenia • Thrombocytopenia	• Platelet function generally returns to normal within 5 days of treatment being received

Active ingredient/ trade names	Indications	Contraindications	Side effects	Comments
Clopidogrel		• Caution: concomitant use of clopidogrel with other oral anticoagulants (bleeding tendency ↑) • Pregnancy/breastfeeding	• Stomach ache • Gastritis • Constipation • Gastrointestinal complaints • Skin rash • Dyspnoea • Rhinitis • Bronchitis, cough • Headache • Dizziness	
Dipyridamole	• In combination with aspirin for the secondary prevention of heart attack • Secondary prevention of ischaemic strokes and transient ischaemic attack (TIAs)	• Hypersensitivity to dipyridamole and aspirin • Severe coronary artery disease (CAD) • Left ventricular outflow obstruction or haemodynamic instability • Existing gastrointestinal ulcers • Abnormally increased bleeding tendency • Pregnancy: 1st and 2nd trimester: strict indication	• Headache, drowsiness, dizziness • Gastrointestinal complaints • Iron deficiency anaemia • Hot flushes	To be taken during or after meals

Active ingredient/ trade names	Indications	Contraindications	Side effects	Comments
Dipyridamole		• Contraindicated in the 3rd trimester • Breastfeeding: strict indication	• Erosive gastritis, gastrointestinal ulcers • Muscle pain • Hypersensitivity reactions	

Lipid-lowering agents Lipid-lowering agents =medicines that lower cholesterol and triglyceride levels in various ways.

Tab. 8 Lipid-lowering agents

Active ingredient/ trade names	Indications	Contraindications	Side effects	Comments
HMG COA reductase inhibitors (statins)				
Atorvastatin Sortis	• Hypercholesterolaemia • Prevention of cardiovascular disease (primary prevention)	The following contraindications apply to **all** statins: • Liver disease • Muscle disorders • Women of childbearing age, due to congenital anomalies associated with statins and pregnancy	The following side effects apply to **all** statins: • Gastrointestinal complaints • Liver damage • Muscle cramps	The following comments apply to **all** statins: • They block the enzyme involved in endogenous cholesterol synthesis thereby lowering cholesterol

Active substance/ trade names	Indications	Contraindications	Side effects	Comments
Pravastatin	• Hypercholesterolaemia • Primary prevention • Secondary prevention • Hyperlipidaemia	• Substantially (by more than 5 times) increased CK values • Pregnancy/breast-feeding	• Muscle pain and cramps • Allergic reactions • Headache, drowsiness, sleep disorders • Back pain • Peripheral oedema • Blood glucose level changes • Hair loss • Liver enzymes ↑	• Treatment with enzyme inhibitors (e.g. ciclosporin), warfarin, gemfibrozil • Do not take with grapefruit juice • To be taken in the evening
Simvastatin	• Hypercholesterolaemia • Cardiovascular prevention			
Ion-exchange resins				
Colestyramine, Lipocol, Merz, Quantalan	• Primary hypercholesterolaemia • Bile acid diarrhoea • Pruritus or jaundice associated with partial biliary obstruction • Can be used in combination with other lipid lowering agents	• Bowel obstruction or biliary obstruction • Constipation	• Gastrointestinal complaints • Allergic reactions • Reduced absorption of fat-soluble vitamins	• To be taken in small doses to start with then gradually increased

Active substance/ trade names	Indications	Contraindications	Side effects	Comments
Fibrates				
Bezafibrate **Fenofibrate**	• Primary hyperlipoproteinaemia: familial hypercholesterolaemia, familial hypertriglyceridaemia, familial combined hyperlipidaemia • Secondary hyperlipidaemia: hypercholesterolaemia	• Gallbladder disease • Patients on dialysis • Pregnancy/breast-feeding • Hepatic failure • Renal failure	• Gastrointestinal complaints • Serum creatinine ↑ • Hypersensitivity reactions • Headache, dizziness • Cholestasis • Photosensitivity • Myotoxicity with muscle pain, weakness and cramps	• Check thyroid function before starting

Oral antidiabetics Oral antidiabetics = medicines used in the treatment of diabetes mellitus that are taken orally.

Tab. 9 Oral antidiabetics

Active ingredient/ trade names	Indications	Contraindications	Side effects	Comments
Glibenclamide **Glimepiride** (Sulphonylureas)	Treatment of type II diabetes mellitus	• Hypersensitivity to sulpho-nylurea, sulphonamides • Type I diabetes • Impaired hepatic and renal function • Diabetic coma • Ketoacidosis • Pregnancy/breastfeeding	• Hypoglycaemia • Gastrointestinal complaints • Allergic skin reactions • Weight gain • Liver enzyme values ↑ • Blood count changes	• β-Blockers, salicylates, coumarins, clofibrate, alcohol have an intensifying effect • To be taken ½ hour before meals
Acarbose	Additional treatment in patients with diabetes mellitus combined with dietary modifica-tions	• Chronic bowel disease • Severe renal failure • Children <18 years	• Bloating • Feeling of fullness	To be taken at the start of meals

Active ingredient/ trade names	Indications	Contraindications	Side effects	Comments
Repaglinide	Treatment of type II diabetes mellitus	• Diabetic ketoacidosis • Children <12 years • Severe hepatic impairment • Pregnancy/breastfeeding	• Hypoglycaemia • Vision problems • Liver enzyme values ↑ • Flulike symptoms • Back pain • Headache • Upper respiratory tract infections	• Effect sets in quickly, duration of effect short → lower risk of hypoglycaemia • Take before meals • Monitor blood glucose closely
Dapaglifozin	Treatment of type II diabetes mellitus	• Diabetic ketoacidosis • Pancreatitis • Pregnancy • Severe renal impairment	• Urinary tract infections • Thrush • Polyuria • Hypotension • Hypoglycaemia	• These drugs inhibit glucose reabsorption • Monitor blood glucose closely
Exanetide	Treatment of type II diabetes mellitus in patients who are already on more than two medications	• Diabetic ketoacidosis • Pancreatitis	• Gastrointestinal complaints	• Glucagon-like peptide-1 (GLP1) agonist – increases insulin secretion given subcutaneously as injections • Moderate weight loss • Monitor blood glucose closely

Active ingredient/ trade names	Indications	Contraindications	Side effects	Comments
Metformin	Treatment of type II diabetes mellitus	• Diabetic ketoacidosis • Severe renal impairment • Cardiac or respiratory failure • Recent heart attack • Hepatic failure	• Gastrointestinal complaints • Headache • Dizziness • Risk of lactic acidosis	• Use in monotherapy or in combination with other antidiabetics or insulin • Tends not to cause weight gain and hypoglycaemia
Gliptins (e.g. linagliptin, sitagliptin)	Treatment of type II diabetes mellitus	• Diabetic ketoacidosis • Acute pancreatitis	• Gastrointestinal upset • Worsening heart failure • Pancreatitis	• These drugs competitively inhibit dipeptidyl peptidase-4 inhibitor (DPP-4) and stimulate insulin secretion • Weight neutral

Insulins   Insulins = blood glucose–lowering hormones that are especially used in the treatment of type I diabetes mellitus.

❗ *Always measure blood glucose in the event of loss of consciousness of unclear origin! Always assume hypoglycaemia. Without current blood glucose values, never give insulin. Instead give glucose and wait for effect.*

❗ *Pay attention to the concentration of insulins! There is U-40 insulin (1 mL ≙ 40 IU insulin, e.g. in ampoules) and U-100 insulin (1 mL ≙ 100 IU insulin, e.g. in pens). Never draw insulin out of a pen with an insulin syringe!*

Tab. 10   Insulins

Type of insulin/ trade names	Injection-meal interval (IMI)	Onset of action	Max. effect	Duration of action
Short-acting insulins				
Regular insulin	15 minutes	After 15–30 minutes	After 2–3 hours	4–6 hours.*
Rapid (short)-acting insulin analogues Lispro Humalog **Aspart** NovoRapid	No IMI, injections also possible after meals	After 10–15 minutes	After 1 hour (corrections possible after 2.5 hours)	2–3 hours.*

Type of insulin/ trade names	Injection-meal interval (IMI)	Onset of action	Max. effect	Duration of action
Long-acting insulins				
Long-acting insulin analogues Insulin glargine Lantus **Insulin Detemir** Levemir	Independent of meals	After 3–4 hours After approx. 3 hours	After 6–14 hours After 4–6 hours	14–24 hours.* 8–10 hours.*
Intermediate-acting insulin	Independent of meals	After 1.5–2 hours	After 4–6 hours	8–12 hours.*
Premixed insulins				
Analogue/protamine premixed insulin (combination of analogue insulin and protamine) With 30% aspart, 70% protamine Novomix 30	No IMI	After 10–15 minutes	After 3–4 hours	6–8 hours.*

*The higher the dose, the longer the total insulin action in direct proportion
**Depending on mixing ratios

Thyroid hormones   Thyroid hormones = thyroid therapeutic agents thyroxine (T_4) and triiodothyronine (T_3).

Thyroid drugs must always be taken approx. ½ hour before meals!

Tab. 11 Thyroid hormones

Active ingredient/ trade names	Indications	Contraindications	Side effects	Comments
L-thyroxine (T_4)	• Hypothyroidism	• Untreated hyperthyroidism • Untreated adrenal failure	• Tachycardia • Palpitations • Anginal pain • Gastrointestinal complaints • Insomnia • Muscle cramps	• Longer plasma half-life (~7 days) than triiodothyronine • Is also easier to control • Take tablets in the morning at least 30 minutes before breakfast
L-thyroxine (T_4)	• Prophylaxis against goitre recurrence following resection of euthyroid goitre • Benign, euthyroid goitre	• Untreated pituitary insufficiency • Acute heart attack • Angina pectoris • Cardiomyopathy	• Side effects especially in the event of an overdose or with an increase in dose that is too rapid	• Treatment in small doses to start with then gradually increased • Often life-long treatment • Soya products can inhibit absorption

Iodized salts   Iodized salts = substances that promote thyroid hormone synthesis when taken in small doses.

Tab. 12 Iodized salts

Active ingredient/ trade names	Indications	Contraindications	Side effects	Comments
Potassium iodide	• Prophylaxis and treatment of euthyroid goitre • Preparation for surgery (when taken in high doses they have an inhibitory effect on thyroid hormone release)	• Overt hyperthyroidism • Iodine allergy • Dermatitis herpetiformis	• Iodine-induced hyperthyroidism • Allergic reactions • If doses are too high: an iatrogenic goitre can be caused	• To be taken after meals
Hyperthyroidism				
Thioureylenes Carbimazole, Propylthiouracil	Treatment of hyperthyroidism	• Large goitre	• Gastrointestinal upset • Rashes • Alopecia • Bone marrow suppression	• Cause inhibition of thyroid perox-idase and reduce thyroid hormone synthesis

Antitussive agents   Antitussive agents = medicines that suppress the cough reflex so that the frequency and intensity of coughing bouts are reduced.

Administer antitussive agents in the evenings so that the patient is able to rest during the night.

Tab. 13   Antitussive agents

Active ingredient/ trade names	Indications	Contraindications	Side effects	Comments
Codeine	Symptomatic treatment of dry cough	Hypersensitivity to codeine Children <12 years	Potential for dependency	Is converted to morphine in the body and so therefore also has an analgesic effect
Noscapine	Short-term, symptomatic treatment of dry cough	Children <16 years		
Noscapine	Unproductive dry cough	• Hypersensitivity to noscapine • Productive cough • Concomitant use of central nervous system (CNS) depressants or alcohol	• Headache, drowsiness • Gastrointestinal complaints • Allergic reactions • Dyspnoea, chest pain	• Bronchospasmolytic effect • No analgesic effect • Acts centrally on the cough centre in the medulla oblongata • May impair attention and responsiveness

Active ingredient/ trade names	Indications	Contraindications	Side effects	Comments
Dextromethorphan	Symptomatic treatment of dry cough	• Asthma/COPD • Pneumonia • Respiratory failure • Concomitant use of monoamine oxidase (MAO) inhibitors • Breastfeeding	• Mild drowsiness • Dizziness • Gastrointestinal complaints • Hypersensitivity reactions	Weak sedative and analgesic effect

Expectorants Expectorants = medicines that promote expectoration, helping to clear mucus from the upper airways. They have the following effects: secretolytic (stimulating the formation of thin mucus), mucolytic (stimulating the thinning of viscous mucus) and/or secretomotor (better removal of mucus through increased movement of cilia).

Tab. 14 Expectorants

Active ingredient/ trade names	Indications	Contraindications	Side effects	Comments
Acetylcysteine (ACC)	For thinning mucus and aiding expectoration in acute and chronic bronchopulmonary disease	• Hypersensitivity to acetylcysteine • Children <1 year: strict indication • Concomitant treatment with antitussive agents should be avoided • Hepatic or renal failure • History of ulcers • Pregnancy/breastfeeding: strict indication	• Gastrointestinal complaints • Allergic reactions • Headache • Tinnitus • Dyspnoea, bronchospasm	• Mucolytic effect • Also used as an antidote for paracetamol poisoning
Carbocisteine	Reduce the viscosity of bronchial secretions, loosening sputum	• Peptic ulceration • Avoid in first trimester of pregnancy	• Rashes	

Diuretics Diuretics = medicines that promote increased production of urine.

❗ *Pay attention to the patient's fluid balance when administering diuretics. Risk of dehydration and deranged electrolytes!*

Tab. 15 Diuretics

Active ingredient/trade names	Indications	Contraindications	Side effects	Comments
Hydrochlorothiazide Esidrix *Note that this medication is only used in combination with other diuretics in the UK.*	• Cardiac, hepatic and renal oedema • Hypertension • Adjuvant symptomatic treatment of chronic heart failure in addition to ACE inhibitors	• Hypersensitivity to hydrochlorothiazide, other thiazides and sulfonamides • Severe renal and hepatic impairment • Acute glomerulonephritis • Hypokalaemia/-natraemia • Hypovolaemia • Hypercalcaemia/-uricaemia • Pregnancy/breastfeeding	• Cardiac arrhythmias • Hyperuricaemia • Hyperglycaemia • Serum lipids ↑ • Fluid and electrolyte imbalance • Thrombocytopenia • Pancreatitis • Gastrointestinal complaints • Orthostatic disorders	• Excretion ↑: sodium, chloride, potassium, magnesium • Excretion ↓: phosphate • Ensure sufficient fluid intake • Increased loss of potassium: give preference to potassium-rich food • This is a thiazide diuretic

Active ingredient/trade names	Indications	Contraindications	Side effects	Comments
Furosemide Lasix	• Oedema • Hypertension • Adjuvant treatment for cerebral oedema • Oliguria due to pre-eclampsia	• Hypersensitivity to furosemide or other sulfonamides • Renal failure with anuria • Hepatic coma and pre-coma • Severe hyponatraemia/-kalaemia • Hypovolaemia • Gout • Hypotension • Breastfeeding • Pregnancy: strict indication	• Electrolyte and metabolic disturbances • Serum uric acid levels ↑ • Thrombocytopenia • Itching, skin and mucous membrane reactions • Gastrointestinal complaints • Metabolic alkalosis • Hyperglycaemia	• Excretion ↑: sodium, chloride, potassium, magnesium, calcium • Potassium-rich diet • Furosemide and torasemide are both loop diuretics
Torasemide Torem	• Hypertension • Treatment and prophylaxis of cardiac oedema and/or effusions due to heart failure	• Renal failure with anuria • Hepatic coma and pre-coma • Severe hyponatraemia/-kalaemia • Hypovolaemia • Gout • Micturition disorders • Cardiac arrhythmias	• Dehydration / hypovolaemia → hypotension, orthostatic disorders, dry mouth, headache, dizziness • Worsening of metabolic alkalosis	

Active ingredient/trade names	Indications	Contraindications	Side effects	Comments
Torasemide		• Concomitant treatment with lithium, aminoglycosides or cephalosporin • Abnormal blood count changes • Children <12 years • Breastfeeding • Pregnancy: strict indication	• Gastrointestinal complaints • Muscle cramps • Allergic reactions • Xerostomia • Serum uric acid levels ↑ • Serum lipids ↑ • Serum glucose ↑ • Certain liver enzymes ↑	
Spironolactone Aldactone	• Primary hyperaldosteronism • Oedema and/or ascites associated with secondary hyperaldosteronism • Can be helpful in the treatment of acne	• Anuria • Acute renal failure • Severe renal failure • Hyperkalaemia • Hyponatraemia • Hypovolaemia or dehydration • Hypotension	• Reversible gynaecomastia in men • Hyperkalaemia • Headache • Sleepiness • Ataxia • Confusion • Uric acid levels ↑ • Thrombocytopenia	• Excretion ↑: sodium, chloride • Excretion ↓: potassium, magnesium • In women: risk of hirsutism and deepening of voice; in men:

Active ingredient/trade names	Indications	Contraindications	Side effects	Comments
Spironolactone			• Antibodies induced by spironolactone • Agranulocytosis • Hypersensitivity reactions	• It works as an antagonist to aldosterone
Triamterene Combination with hydrochlorothiazide	• Hypertension • Oedema	• Severe renal impairment • Renal failure with anuria • Hepatic coma and pre-coma • Severe hyponatraemia/-kalaemia • Hypovolaemia • Hyperkalaemia/-calcaemia • Diabetes mellitus • Gout • Pregnancy/breastfeeding	• Fluid and electrolyte imbalance • Hyperuricaemia • Gastrointestinal complaints • Hypotension, orthostatic regulatory disorders • Muscle pain/cramps • Dry mouth, thirst, feeling of dizziness • Headache • Hyperglycaemia • Vision problems	• Excretion ↑: sodium, chloride • Excretion ↓: potassium, magnesium • Caution when wearing contact lenses as impaired tear formation

Active ingredient/trade names	Indications	Contraindications	Side effects	Comments
Amiloride	• Hypertension • Cardiac oedema • Hepatic oedema	• Severe renal impairment • Acute glomerulonephritis • Hepatic coma and pre-coma • Severe hyponatraemia/-kalaemia • Hypovolaemia • Hyperkalaemia/-calcaemia • Gout • Concomitant treatment with other potassium-sparing medicines or potassium salts • Breastfeeding • Pregnancy: strict indication	• Blood count changes • Fluid and electrolyte imbalance • Acid alkaline imbalance • Hyperuricaemia • Hyperglycaemia • Hypersensitivity reactions • Dry mouth, thirst, feeling of weakness/dizziness • Depression, insomnia, nervousness, restlessness • Vision problems • Dyspnoea, breathing difficulties • Gastrointestinal complaints • Anginal pain, ECG changes	

Antiemetic agents   Antiemetic agents = medicines that suppress nausea and vomiting.
Administer antiemetic agents early enough before food so that the patient can eat.

Tab. 16 Antiemetic agents

Active ingredient/trade names	Indications	Contraindications	Side effects	Comments
Metoclopramide (MCP) Paspertin	Nausea, urge to vomit, vomiting (following chemotherapy, as a result of radiotherapy or symptomatic)	• Hypersensitivity to metoclopramide • Phaeochromocytoma • Prolactin-dependent tumours • Mechanical bowel obstruction • Gastrointestinal perforation • Gastrointestinal bleeding • Epilepsy • Extrapyramidal symptoms • Children <1 year	• Diarrhoea • Constipation • Fatigue • Headache • Dizziness • Anxiety, restlessness	• To be taken approx. 30 minutes before meals • Prolonged use carries the increased risk of movement disorders → treatment should not exceed 3 months
Cyclizine	• Nausea and vomiting • Motion sickness and vertigo	• Severe heart failure • Neuromuscular disorder • Epilepsy • Prostatic hypertrophy	• Hypertension • Drowsiness • Headache • Dry mouth • Blurred vision • Gastrointestinal complaints	Can be given orally, i.m. or i.v.

Active ingredient/trade names	Indications	Contraindications	Side effects	Comments
Domperidone Motilium	• Motility disorders of the upper gastrointestinal tract • Nausea, urge to vomit, vomiting	• Hypersensitivity to domperidone • Prolactin-dependent tumours • Mechanical bowel obstruction • Gastrointestinal bleeding • Children <12 years	• Gastrointestinal complaints • Prolactin increase, gynaecomastia, galactorrhoea, menstrual disorders	• To be taken 15–30 minutes before meals • In the event of overdose: there is no specific antidote • Length of treatment: usually max. 10 days
Ondansetron	• Used in the treatment of nausea and vertigo • Useful for patients having chemotherapy or anaesthetic preoperatively	• Congenital long QT syndrome	• Constipation • Flushing • Hiccups	• Monitor QT interval with regular ECGs

Antiulcerants   Antiulcerants = medicines used in the treatment of gastric and duodenal ulcers.

Tab. 17 Antiulcerants

Active ingredient/trade names	Indications	Contraindications	Side effects	Comments
Omeprazole	• Heartburn • Gastric and duodenal ulcers	• Hypersensitivity to omeprazole • Use of nelfinavir (against HIV)	• Headache • Nausea • Constipation • Diarrhoea	Is a proton pump inhibitor
Ranitidine Ranitic	• Duodenal ulcers • Reflux oesophagitis • Zollinger-Ellison syndrome	Hypersensitivity to ranitidine	• Headache • Nausea • Constipation • Diarrhoea	• Is one of the H_2-receptor blockers • Effect weaker than with proton pump inhibitors

Antidiarrhoeal agents   Antidiarrhoeal agents = medicines used to treat diarrhoea.

Tab. 18 Antidiarrhoeal agents

Active ingredient/trade names	Indications	Contraindications	Side effects	Comments
Activated charcoal	• Acute diarrhoea • Oral poisoning	• Diarrhoea with fever • Poisoning with corrosive substances	• After very high doses: constipation leading to ileus	

Active ingredient/trade names	Indications	Contraindications	Side effects	Comments
Activated charcoal			• Can inhibit effects of other medicines	• Black stool
Loperamide Imodium	Diarrhoea due to motility disorders	• Conditions where slow bowel movements are to be avoided • Antibiotic-associated colitis • Hepatic dysfunction • Diarrhoea of infectious origin (apart from mild travel diarrhoea without fever, with no bloody stool) • Children <2 years	• Gastrointestinal complaints • Headache • Constipation • Stomach cramps, nausea • Hypersensitivity reactions • Drowsiness, fatigue, dry mouth	If there is no improvement 48 hours after start of treatment in the case of acute diarrhoea, the medicine should be discontinued

Laxatives   Laxatives = purgatives; medicines used to accelerate the movement of food through the gastrointestinal tract and help empty the bowel.

Drink a lot of fluids and move around a lot as a first step to combat constipation.

Tab. 19 Laxatives

Active ingredient/trade names	Indications	Contraindications	Side effects	Comments
Lactulose	• Constipation, constipation prophylaxis • Conditions that necessitate ease of bowel movement • Cirrhosis of the liver (prevention and treatment of ammonia poisoning)	• Lactose and/or fructose intolerance • Ileus • Acute inflammatory gastrointestinal disease • Water and electrolyte imbalance	• Stomach ache, cramps, flatulence • Nausea, vomiting • Prolonged use causes water and electrolyte imbalance	• Onset of action: 2–10 hours after intake • In the event of diabetes mellitus: take content of fructose and lactose into account • With prolonged use: monitor potassium
Sorbitol Rectal use in enemas: Microlax	• Constipation • Conditions that necessitate ease of bowel movement • Used as bowel preparation prior to bowel investigation	• Ileus • Hereditary fructose intolerance • Bleeding around the anus • Diverticulitis • Bowel perforation • Children <6 years	Loss of water and minerals	Effect sets in after a few minutes

Active ingredient/trade names	Indications	Contraindications	Side effects	Comments
Linseed Linusit linseed	• Constipation • Irritable bowel syndrome	• Ileus • Pronounced hyperlipidaemia	• Bloating • Ileus caused by adhesions, if no sufficient fluid intake	• Several teaspoons several times a day • Crush linseed beforehand • Onset of action after several days • Sufficient fluid intake required • Interval for taking other medicines: 0.5–1 hour
Polyethylene glycol, e.g., Macrogol 4000	Chronic constipation in adults, short- and long-term treatment of constipation	• Hypersensitivity to Macrogol • Existing or impending bowel obstruction or perforation • Toxic megacolon • Inflammatory bowel disease	• Feeling of fullness, flatulence, nausea, diarrhoea, vomiting • Headache, dizziness • Hypersensitivity reactions	• Interval for taking other medicines: at least 2 hours • Is absorbed in small amounts, therefore it is safe to use in pregnancy

Active ingredient/trade names	Indications	Contraindications	Side effects	Comments
Bisacodyl Dulcolax	• Short-term treatment of constipation • Conditions that necessitate ease of bowel movement	• Hypersensitivity to bisacodyl • Ileus • Acute inflammation of the gastrointestinal tract (e.g., appendicitis) • Children <2 years	• Stomach ache • If used for too long or too frequently • Water/electrolyte imbalance (particularly K^+ ↓ →muscle weakness, cardiac arrhythmias) • Diarrhoea	• Do not use for more than 1 week • Should not be taken orally with milk • Onset of action perorally: 6–8 hours, rectally: 0.5–1 hour
Sodium picosulfate Laxoberal		• Hypersensitivity to sodium picosulfate • Ileus • Acute inflammation of the gastrointestinal tract (e.g., appendicitis) • Children <4 years		• Onset of action: after approx. 8 hours • If used in drop form exact dosage and tapering possible

Active ingredient/trade names	Indications	Contraindications	Side effects	Comments
Senna glycoside Agiolax	Short-term treatment of constipation	• Hypersensitivity to senna glycoside and other combination ingredients • Excessive hardening of stool: enteroliths, fecal impaction • Ileus • Acute inflammation of the gastrointestinal tract (e.g., Crohn disease, ulcerative colitis, appendicitis) • Children <10 years	• If used for too long or too frequently • Water/electrolyte imbalance (particularly K^+ ↓ →muscle weakness, cardiac arrhythmias) • Slow transit ↑ • Diarrhoea • Albuminuria • Haematuria	• Onset of action: 8–10 hours after intake • Interval for taking other medicines: 0.5–1 hour • (Harmless) red discolouration of urine possible
Glycerol Rectal use	• Constipation • Painful defecation	• Hypersensitivity to glycerine • Ileus • Appendicitis	Local irritation	• Specially formulated suppositories for children • Low-dose use in infants possible

Antispasmodic (spasmolytic) agents Antispasmodic (spasmolytic) agents = antispasmodic drugs.

Tab. 20 Antispasmodic (spasmolytic) agents

Active ingredient/trade names	Indications	Contraindications	Side effects	Comments
Parasympatholytic agents				
Hyoscine butylbromide Buscopan	• Abdominal pain caused by spasms • Stomach cramps • Irritable bowel syndrome	• Hypersensitivity to butylbromide • Myasthenia gravis • Megacolon • i.v.: untreated narrow angle glaucoma, prostatic hypertrophy with urinary retention, gastrointestinal stricture, tachycardia • Pregnancy/breastfeeding: strict indication • Children <6 years	• Constipation • Diarrhoea • Skin reactions • Saliva production ↓ • Urinary retention • Dizziness, fatigue • i.v.: tachycardia, BP ↓, accommodation disorders	Slow i.m. or i.v.: administration, to be performed by the doctor only. More commonly prescribed orally
Neurotropic and musculotropic antispasmodic (spasmolytic) drugs				
Mebeverine Duspatal	Irritable bowel syndrome	• Hypersensitivity to mebeverine • Severe hepatic impairment • Paralytic ileus • Children <18 years	• Headache, dizziness • Fatigue • Allergic reactions • Loss of appetite	To be taken with plenty of water 20 minutes before meals

Antibiotics Antibiotics = medicines that are effective against bacteria. They inhibit the growth of bacteria (bacteriostasis) or kill them (bactericidal activity).

Tab. 21 Antibiotics

Active ingredient/trade names	Indications	Contraindications	Side effects*	Comments**
Ampicillin Ampicillin	• ENT infections • Lower respiratory tract infections including pertussis (whooping cough) • Respiratory and ENT infections	• Beta-lactam allergy • Allergies to penicillin	• Gastrointestinal complaints • Exanthema	• Check for penicillin allergy before giving this antibiotic

Active ingredient/trade names	Indications	Contraindications	Side effects*	Comments**
Amoxicillin Amoxypen	• Infections of the kidneys and urinary tract • Gastrointestinal infections • Skin and soft tissue infections • Biliary or urinary tract infections (e.g., with enterococci) • Salmonella infections • Listeriosis • Endocarditis prophylaxis • Typhoid fever • Osteitis, osteomyelitis	• Allergy to penicillin • Infectious mono-nucleosis (can cause widespread rash)	• Allergic reactions (local or generalised) • Drug fever • Taste alteration • Dry mouth • Fungal infections • Dizziness, headache • Myoclonus, seizures • Gastrointestinal upset	• Interactions possible: digoxin, allopurinol, anticoagulants, methotrexate, hormonal contraceptives • Broad-spectrum antibiotic

Active ingredient/trade names	Indications	Contraindications	Side effects*	Comments**
Penicillin G	• ENT infections • Lower respiratory tract infections • Gynaecological infections • Actinomycosis • Endocarditis • Erysipelas, gas gangrene • Osteomyelitis • Peritonitis • Septicaemia • Tetanus • Wound infections • Meningococcal meningitis	• Beta-lactam allergy	• Dose-dependent neutropenia • Allergic reactions (local and/or generalized → anaphylaxis) • Exanthema, local reactions in the case of i.v. administration	• Ask patients if they are allergic to penicillin before administering • Use particularly in the event of infections that are caused by streptococci, pneumococci, gonococci, meningococci, or spirochaetes • Broad-spectrum antibiotic
Flucloxacillin	Streptococci and staphylococci producing infections: • Sepsis • Cellulitis • Endocarditis • Ostemoyeltiis • Mastitis • Respiratory tract • ENT infection • Post-operative wound • Abscesses of skin/soft tissue	• History of hepatic impairment • Serious underlying illness • Penicillin allergy	• Gastrointestinal disorders • Vein irritation (in the case of i.v. administration) • Exanthema • Drug fever • Taste alteration • Dry mouth • Glossitis, stomatitis	• Ask patient if allergic to penicillin • Can be given orally or intravenously depending on severity of the infection • Broad-spectrum antibiotic

Active ingredient/trade names	Indications	Contraindications	Side effects*	Comments**
Flucloxacillin			• Laryngeal oedema • Liver function readings temporarily ↑ • Blood count changes	
Piperacillin Piperacillin in combination with tazobactam - known as Tazocin	• Sepsis • Endocarditis • Peritonitis • Lower respiratory tract infection • Gastrointestinal infections • Biliary tract infections • Infections of the kidneys and urinary tract • Infections of the reproductive organs without gonorrhoea • Gynaecological infections • Infections of bone and soft tissue • Infection prophylaxis in at-risk patients • Tazobactam is often used in the treatment of neutropenic sepsis	• Hypersensitivity to piperacillin • Beta-lactam allergy • Patients prone to allergic response • Pregnancy/breast-feeding (avoid unless benefit outweighs risk)	• Allergic reactions, drug fever • Gastrointestinal complaints • Exanthema, itching • Bilirubin ↑ • Transaminases ↑ • Vein irritation (thrombo-phlebitis) • Headache • Joint pain • Taste disorders • Coagulation disorders • Leukopenia even leading to agranulocytosis (if used for >10 days)	• Ask patient if allergic to penicillin • Broad-spectrum antibiotic

Active ingredient/trade names	Indications	Contraindications	Side effects*	Comments**
Cefuroxime	• Acute and chronic infections of the respiratory tract, reproductive organs, bones, skin, and soft tissue • Urinary tract infections • Acute uncomplicated gonorrhoea • ENT infections • Sepsis	• Hypersensitivity to cefuroxime	• Allergic reactions • Drug fever • Creatinine ↑ and urea ↑ in serum • i.v. administration: inflammatory irritation of the vein wall • i.m. injection: pain, indurations at the infection site	• Ask patient if allergic to penicillin (cross-sensitivity) • Reduced effectiveness of hormonal contraceptives
Erythromycin	• Legionnaire's disease and other respiratory diseases • Severe forms of acne • Erysipelas • Scarlet fever • Diphtheria • Urethritis	• Hypersensitivity to erythromycin and other macrolides • QT interval prolongation	• Vein irritation • Gastrointestinal complaints • Liver enzymes ↑ • QT interval prolongations • Allergic skin reactions • Angio-oedema • Joint swelling, drug fever • Transient CNS side effects	• Check for erythomycin allergies before administering

Active ingredient/trade names	Indications	Contraindications	Side effects*	Comments**
Erythromycin	• Gonorrhoea • Syphilis	• In particular hypokalaemia and hypomagnesaemia • Bradycardia and other cardiac arrhythmias	• Intrahepatic cholestasis and cholestatic jaundice particularly when used repeatedly or for more than 10 days	
Clarithromycin	• Respiratory tract infections • ENT infections • Skin infections	• Hypersensitivity to clarithromycin and other macrolides • First trimester of pregnancy • Breastfeeding: avoid unless benefit outweighs risk	• Vein irritation • Gastrointestinal complaints • Temporary impairment of smell and taste • Candidiasis • Upper abdominal complaints • Headache	• Need to reduce the dose in renal impairment • Check for allergy before administering

Active ingredient/trade names	Indications	Contraindications	Side effects*	Comments**
Imipenem with cilastatin	• Severe abdominal infections • Sepsis with unclear pathogens • Severe nosocomial infections • Mixed infections with aerobes or anaerobes	• Hypersensitivity to imipenem or other carbapenems (if a person has a beta-lactam allergy there may be cross-sensitivity!) • Pregnancy and breastfeeding: avoid unless benefit outweighs risk	• Local reactions, vein inflammation • Prolonged prothrombin time • Increase in liver enzymes • Gastrointestinal complaints • Blood count changes • Skin reactions • Severe allergic general reactions • Renal impairment • Seizure threshold ↓	• Antibiotic of last resort • Not indicated for meningitis • Very broad spectrum
Gentamicin Refobacin	Severe infections, particularly in combination with immune deficiency, e.g., • Urogenital infections (with the exception of gonorrhoea and syphilis) • Nosocomial pneumonia • Endocarditis	• Hypersensitivity to the active ingredient or other aminoglycosides • Only in the event of a life-threatening situation if there is pre-existing sensorineural hearing loss	• Allergy • Gastrointestinal disorders • Headache • Nephro- and ototoxicity • Hearing damage • Vestibular damage	

Active ingredient/trade names	Indications	Contraindications	Side effects*	Comments**
Gentamicin	• Intra-abdominal infections • Nosocomial sepsis • Meningitis as a result of gram-negative pathogens • Osteomyelitis and septic arthritis	• Advanced renal failure, previous neuromuscular disease, concomitant muscle relaxant administration • Pregnancy: contraindicated in the 1st trimester, then only if benefit outweighs risk	• Blood count changes • Electrolyte changes • Liver enzymes ↑ • Respiratory depression	• Severe infections with gram-negative pathogens, hospital-acquired infections, and in immunocompromised patients • Risk of falls and hardness of hearing • Most commonly given i.v. • Check renal function prior to prescribing and administering

Active ingredient/trade names	Indications	Contraindications	Side effects*	Comments**
Ciprofloxacin Ciprobay	• Lower respiratory tract infections caused by gram-negative bacteria • Chronic suppurative otitis media • Acute exacerbation of chronic sinusitis • Urinary tract infections • Pelvic inflammatory disease including infections as a result of *Neisseria gonorrhoea* • Gastrointestinal infections • Infections of the skin and soft tissue • Bone and joint infections • Gonococcal urethritis and cervicitis • Intra-abdominal infections • Infection prophylaxis in at-risk patients	• Hypersensitivity to ciprofloxacin or other quinolines • Concomitant use with tizanidine • Epilepsy: use with caution as quinolones can precipitate seizures • Pregnancy: should be avoided if possible because it can cause arthropathy	• Gastrointestinal complaints • Fungal infections • Dizziness • Skin reactions • Headache, drowsiness, sleep disorders • Restlessness, psychomotor hyperactivity • Psychotic reactions • Allergy • Blood count changes • Joint pain • Renal impairment • Non-specific pain, general malaise • Tendon rupture, particularly affecting the Achilles tendon	• May impair performance of driving • Quinolone-type antibiotic

Active ingredient/trade names	Indications	Contraindications	Side effects*	Comments**
Clindamycin Sobelin	• Infections of the bones and joints and skin and soft tissue • ENT infections • Infections of the teeth and jaw • Lower respiratory tract infections • Infections of the pelvis and abdomen • Acne • Septicaemia • Endocarditis	• Allergy to clindamycin and lincomycin (cross-sensitivity) • Gastrointestinal disease • Severe hepatic impairment • Disorders of neuromuscular transmission	• Allergy • Gastrointestinal complaints • Exanthema • Reversible blood count changes • Serum transaminases temporarily ↑ • Neuromuscular blockade • Vein irritation in the case of i.v. administration	• In combination with vitamin K antagonists, there is an increase in the anticoagulation effect. Need to monitor INR closely.
Cotrimoxazole	• Upper and lower respiratory tract infections • *Pneumocystis jiroveci pneumonia* • ENT infections (apart from strep throat) • Uncomplicated cystitis in women	• Hypersensitivity to sulfonamide or trimethoprim • Erythema multiforme • Congenital glucose-6-dehydrognase	• Gastrointestinal upset • Fungal infections • Hyperkalaemia • Headache • Allergic reactions	Teratogenic in first trimester of pregnancy; therefore avoid

Active ingredient/trade names	Indications	Contraindications	Side effects*	Comments**
Cotrimoxazole	• Urinary tract infections • Long-term relapse prevention for urinary tract infections • Infections of the female and male genital tract • Granuloma inguinale • Infections of the gastrointestinal tract (shigellosis, traveller's diarrhoea, chronic carriers of typhoid fever) • Nocardiosis • Brucellosis	• Deficiency affecting red blood cells, haemoglobin abnormalities • Severe renal or hepatic impairment • Acute porphyria • Pre-term infants • Neonates with hyperbilirubinaemia or glucose-6-dehydrogenase deficiency affecting red blood cells • Osteomyelitis, caused by staphylococci • Pregnancy (teratogenic in 1st trimester and neonatal haemolysis in 3rd trimester)	• Rarely: blood count changes • Increased K^+	Use a reduced dose in renal impairment

Active ingredient/trade names	Indications	Contraindications	Side effects*	Comments**
Metronidazole	• Infections of the gastrointestinal tract • ENT infections • Lower respiratory tract infections • Anaerobic infections • Used in the eradication of *H. pylori* (gastrointestinal ulcers) • Brain abscesses • Osteomyelitis • Endocarditis • Infections of the female genital area • Infections of the teeth, mouth, and jaw area • Infection prophylaxis • Trichomoniasis • Amoebiasis • Giardiasis • Moderate rosacea • Bacterial vaginosis	• Hypersensitivity to metronidazole • Pregnancy: 1st trimester	• Gastrointestinal complaints • Metallic taste, coating of the tongue • Glossitis, stomatitis • Dysuria, urinary incontinence • Yeast-like fungal infections in the genital area • Sleepiness, insomnia • Confusion, irritability • Vision problems • Allergic reactions • Headache • Ataxia, seizures	• Patient must abstain from alcohol • Should generally not exceed a treatment duration of 10 days • Dark urine (harmless)

*Gastrointestinal complaints (nausea, vomiting) with all antibiotics, rarely pseudomembranous colitis.
**Examinations arranged by medics (e.g., blood tests) also take place.

Antiviral agents Antiviral agents = medicines that disrupt normal cell function, thereby inhibiting virus replication.

Tab. 22 Antiviral agents

Active ingredient/trade names	Indications	Contraindications	Side effects	Comments
Aciclovir Zovirax	• Herpes simplex • Herpes zoster (shingles)	• Hypersensitivity to aciclovir (valaciclovir) • Impaired renal function, anuria • Severe disorders of the immune system	• Hypersensitivity reactions • Gastrointestinal disorders • Dizziness, headache	• Preferably use with the first signs of herpes • Do not apply to mucous membranes—risk of local irritation
Oseltamivir Tamiflu	Treatment and post-exposure prophylaxis of influenza	• Hypersensitivity to oseltamivir • Severe renal impairment • Pregnancy/breastfeeding	• Gastrointestinal disorders • Insomnia, drowsiness • Cough, bronchitis	• Only effective against influenza viruses • Does not replace flu vaccine!

Antimycotic (antifungal) agents Antimycotic (antifungal) agents = medicines used in the treatment of fungal infections. These are either indicated for local or systemic use.

Tab. 23 Antimycotic (antifungal) agents

Active ingredient/ trade names	Indications	Contraindications	Side effects	Comments
Amorolfine Loceryl	Onchomycoses caused by dermato-phytes, yeasts, and mould	Hypersensitivity to amorolfine	• Nausea, vomiting, diarrhoea • Fever • Anaemia • Skin rash • Headache • Liver enzyme values ↑	Local
Bifonazole	• Mycoses of the skin • Infections as a result of *Corynebac-terium minutissimum* • Thrush (treatment with canesten containing clotrimazole)	Hypersensitivity to bifonazole		Local
Caspofungin Cancidas	• Aspergillosis • Invasive candidiasis • Particularly fungal infections in the event of fever and neutropenia	Hypersensitivity to caspofungin		Parenteral
Nystatin	Nystatin-sensitive yeast infections	Hypersensitivity to nystatin or a related substance		Peroral

Antiallergic agents Antiallergic agents = substances with antiallergic effect which suppress the symptoms of allergic disease or prevent it from developing.

Tab. 24 Antiallergic agents

Active ingredient/ trade names	Indications	Contraindications	Side effects	Comments
Antihistamines (histamine antagonists, histamine receptor blockers)				
Cetirizine	Symptomatic relief of allergy (hay fever, chronic idio-pathic urticarial)	• Severe liver disease • Epilepsy • Prostatic hypertrophy	• Drowsiness • Palpitations • Urinary retention • Dry mouth • Blurred vision	Should be avoided in acute porphyrias
Mast cell stabilisers (mediator release inhibltors)				
Sodium cromoglicate	Chronic obstructive pulmo-nary disease bronchiectasis	Hypersensitivity to cromoglicic acid	Local irritation	Local use (e.g., nasal spray, eye drops, metered-dose inhaler)
Glucocorticoids				
Mometasone	• Inhaled: asthma • Nasal: allergic rhinitis	• Untreated bacterial, fungal or viral skin lesions	• Burning, itching • If used topically: paraesthe-sia, folliculitis	• Occurrence of further side effects if used long term • Do not use in the eye area

Active ingredient/ trade names	Indications	Contraindications	Side effects	Comments
Mometasone			• pharyngitis, changes in voice	
Prednisolone, methyl- prednisolone	Used in inflammatory conditions (e.g., acute asthma, cancer, immunosuppression in patients with transplants, rheumatological conditions, and inflammatory bowel disease)	Caution starting antibiotics if the patient has an infection and ensure the patient has been screened for dormant bacteria/viruses (e.g., TB or HIV)	• Adrenal suppression • Diabetes mellitus • Osteoporosis • Muscle wasting • Peptic ulceration • Acne • Skin thinning	• Glucocorticosteroids can be prescribed topically, orally, per rectum, or intravenously depending on the use of the steroid • Need to consider gastric ulcer protection and bone protection if prescribing long courses of steroids • Check blood sugars regularly whilst on prednisolone

Analgesics Analgesics = pain medication, painkillers; pain-relieving or pain-killing medicines.
Use pain scale to assess pain.

Tab. 25 Analgesics

Active ingredient/ trade names	Indications	Contraindications	Side effects	Comments
Non-opioid analgesics				
Paracetamol	• Moderate, non-visceral pain • Fever	• Hypersensitivity • Severe liver and kidney damage • Risk of suicide	• Nausea • Allergic reactions • Renal impairment • Liver damage	• Orally/as a supp.: 0.5–1 g up to 4× daily • i.v.: 1 g up to 4× daily
Aspirin Aspirin	• Pain • Bone metastases • Fever • Inflammation • Platelet aggregation inhibition • Treatment of an acute myocardial infarction and stroke	• Intolerance • Stomach ulcers • Asthma • Haemorrhagic diathesis • Anticoagulant treatment	• Gastrointestinal intolerance (bleeding, ulcer) • Allergic reaction • Asthma attacks	• Orally: up to 3 g daily, single dose: 0.5–1 g

Active ingredient/ trade names	Indications	Contraindications	Side effects	Comments
Ibuprofen	• Fever • Pain • Rheumatism • Gout	• Stomach or bowel ulcers • Severe liver or kidney damage • Blood coagulation disorders • Pregnancy	• Gastrointestinal complaints • Bronchoconstriction • CNS disorders (including depression, fatigue) • Allergic reaction	• Pain: 200–400 mg p.o. up to 3× daily • Rheumatism: max. 800 mg p.o. up to 3× daily
Diclofenac	• Rheumatism • Pain and inflammation • Gout	• → Ibuprofen • Cardiovascular disease	→ Ibuprofen	Always administer with gastric protection
Opioid analgesics				
Dihydrocodeine prolonged-release DHC 60/90/120	Moderately severe pain	• Hypersensitivity • Respiratory failure • Acute asthma attack • Chronic and acute pancreatitis • Increased intracranial pressure	• Constipation • Dyspnoea • Nausea, vomiting • Dizziness, drowsiness • Sedation • Dry mouth	Not subject to controlled drug prescription
Naloxone	Severe and very severe pain	• Hypersensitivity • Opiate dependency • Pronounced hepatic failure • Children <2 years	→ Dihydrocodeine	Not subject to controlled drug prescription

Active ingredient/ trade names	Indications	Contraindications	Side effects	Comments
Tramadol Ultram	Moderately severe to severe pain	• Acute poisoning with alcohol • Epilepsy • Pre-treatment with MAO inhibitors • Impaired respiratory function • Children <25 kg	→ Dihydrocodeine	Not subject to controlled drug prescription
Morphine MST, Sevredol, Zomorph or Oramorph	Long-term pain treatment for tumour pain and other severe and very severe pain	• Ileus • Acute abdomen • Known hypersensitivity	• → Dihydrocodeine • Headache • Erythema, itching • Sweating • Micturition disorders	Subject to controlled drug prescription
Buprenorphine Butrans	Severe and very severe pain	• Opioid dependency • Severe respiratory failure • Severe hepatic failure • Use of MAO inhibitors	• → Dihydrocodeine • Headache • Erythema, itching • Sweating	• Subject to controlled drug prescription • Used most frequently as patches

Active ingredient/ trade names	Indications	Contraindications	Side effects	Comments
Fentanyl	• Tumour pain • Acute or chronic severe pain	• Bradyarrhythmias • Severely impaired CNS function	• Acute anaphylactic reactions • Dependency • Withdrawal symptoms after sudden discontinuation (nausea, vomiting, shivering)	Subject to controlled drug prescription, patches cannot be divided

Hypnotic agents   Hypnotic agents = sleep-inducing medicines.

Tab. 26   Hypnotic agents

Active ingredient/ trade names	Indications	Contraindications	Side effects	Comments
Benzodiazepines				
Midazolam	• Problems in getting to sleep (sleep-onset insomnia) (short-term use) • Premedication for anaesthesia • Used in the treatment of prolonged seizures	• Problems of dependency • Acute drug or alcohol intoxication • Severe respiratory failure • Severe hepatic failure • Sleep apnoea • Depressive disorders • Concomitant treatment with ketoconazole, itraconazole, voriconazole, HIV protease inhibitors • Breastfeeding • Pregnancy/birth: strict indication • Myasthenia gravis	• Potential for dependency • Morning fatigue • Impairment in concentration and responsiveness • Headache • Muscle relaxation → risk of falls and accidents • Subdued emotions • Respiratory depression • Vision problems • Libido changes • Floppy infant syndrome (muscle weakness in neonates) • Paradoxical reactions (restlessness, insomnia)	• Short duration of action (half-life <5 hours) • Disadvantage: night-time awakening or withdrawal insomnia

Active ingredient/ trade names	Indications	Contraindications	Side effects	Comments
Temazepam Planum	• Problems in getting to sleep (sleep-onset insomnia) and problems in staying asleep (sleep-maintenance insomnia) (short-term use) • Diazepam is used in the treatment of prolonged seizures	→ Midazolam	→ Midazolam	• Medium-length duration of action (half-life: 5–24 hours) • Disadvantage: risk of accumulation, after-effect
Brotizolam Lendormin				
Lormetazepam Noctamid				
Nitrazepam Radedorm				• Long duration of action (half-life: 20–50 hours)
Diazepam Valium				
Oxazepam Adumbran	Short-term use for: • Sleep disorders • Anxiety disorders • States of stress, agitation	→ Midazolam	→ Midazolam	Medium-length duration of action (half-life: 5–15 hours)

Active ingredient/ trade names	Indications	Contraindications	Side effects	Comments
Lorazepam Tavor	• Symptomatic short-term treatment of states of stress, agitation, and anxiety • Sedative before diagnostic procedures or surgery • Sleep disorders • Termination of prolonged seizures	• Problems of dependency • Acute drug or alcohol intoxication • Myasthenia gravis • Impaired respiratory function • Children <6 years • Elderly and depressive patients: strict indication • Pregnancy/breastfeeding: strict indication	→ Midazolam	Medium-length duration of action (half-life: 10–18 hours)
Benzodiazepine-like substances				
Zolpidem Stilnox **Zopiclone** Ximovan	Short-term treatment of sleep disorders	• Severe hepatic or respiratory impairment • Sleep apnoea • Myasthenia gravis • Pregnancy/breastfeeding • Children/adolescents < 18 years	• Dependency possible with prolonged use • Sleepiness, drowsiness the following day • Gastrointestinal complaints • Vision problems • Paradoxical reactions	Impairs ability to drive and react No alcohol!

Antidepressants Antidepressants = psychopharmaceuticals that are used to treat affective disorders.

! *Anti depressant drugs can have a delayed beneficial effect and sometimes worsen mood and increase the risk of suicide intiially.*

Tab. 27 Antidepressants

Active ingredient/ trade names	Indications	Contraindications	Side effects	Comments
Acute treatment				
Fluoxetine Prozac	• Depression • Anxiety and obsessive compulsive disorder	• Epilepsy • Acute mania • Combination with MAO inhibitors	• Nausea, vomiting, diarrhoea • Agitation, sleep disorders • Sexual dysfunction	• 20 up to max. 80 mg daily, dose reduction (withdrawal symptoms!) • Cannot be stopped abruptly, must be titrated down • It is a selective serotonin reuptake inhibitor

Active ingredient/ trade names	Indications	Contraindications	Side effects	Comments
Venlafaxine	• Depression • Generalized anxiety disorders	Children <18 years		• 2 × 75 mg daily up to max. 225 mg daily, dose reduction (withdrawal symptoms!), if necessary, monitor cholesterol values • Cannot be stopped abruptly, must be titrated down • It is a selective serotonin-norepinephrine reuptake inhibitor
Mirtazapine Remergil	• Depression • Anxiety	Children <18 years	• Sedation • Weight gain • Orthostatic hypotension	• Maintenance dose: 15–45 mg daily p.o., 6 up to max. 21 mg daily i.v. • Cannot be stopped abruptly, must be titrated down
Carbamazepine	Effective treatment of bipolar affective disorder and epilepsy	• Acute porphyria • Bone marrow suppression • Cardiac conduction abnormalities	• Drowsiness • Nausea • Headache • Rashes • Ataxia • Bone marrow suppression	• GABA agonist • Has multiple drug interactions due to induction of hepatic enzymes

Active ingredient/ trade names	Indications	Contraindications	Side effects	Comments
Lithium	• Alternative antidepressant • Used in the treatment of mania, bipolar disorder, and recurrent depression	• Renal impairment • Cardiovascular disease • Hyponatraemia • Pregnancy: particularly the 1st trimester (cardiac abnormalities of fetus) • Thyroid dysfunction	• Weight gain • Tremor • Polyuria, polydipsia • Na^+ and K^+ loss • Goitre/thyroid dysfunction • Cardiomyopathy	• Narrow therapeutic index (monitor blood values) • Not for children <12 years! • May lower seizure threshold
Olanzapine Clozaapine	Treatment of schizophrenia and acute mania	• Acute heart attack • Narrow angle glaucoma • Pyloric stenosis	• Diabetes mellitus • Weight gain • Extrapyramidal side effects • Anti-cholinergic effects • Bone marrow suppression	Clozapine is usually given as a last resort because of rare but severe neutropenia

Active ingredient/ trade names	Indications	Contraindications	Side effects	Comments
Atypical antipsychotics Risperidone, Aripiprazole, Quetiapine	• Treatment of schizophrenia • Bipolar disorder • Psychosis • Severe delirium/ agitation (short term)	• Hyperprolactinaemia • Children <5 years • Intoxication with alcohol • Lewy body dementia	• Prolactin increase • Change in blood glucose and lipids • Weight gain • Parkinsonism (extra-pyramidal signs) • Fatigue • Raised lipid and glucose levels	• Initial dose: 2 mg daily, maintenance dose depending on the severity of the illness • Given orally or i.m. (longer acting) • Atypical anti-psychotic

Parkinson's disease

Active ingredient/trade names	Indications	Contraindications	Side effects	Comments
Levo-Dopa (dopamine precursor)	Treatment of Parkinson's disease	Closed angle glaucoma	• Nausea and vomiting • Psychosis • Hypotension • Dyskinesia	Larger doses are more likely to result in adverse effects
Selegiline, Entacapone	Treatment of Parkinson's disease (used in conjunction with Levo-dopa to reduce end of dose fluctuations)	Caution in liver impairment	• Dry mouth • Dyspepsia • Headache • Depression • Abnormal dreams	• Monoamine oxidase B inhibitors • Cannot stop these drugs abruptly
Ropinirole, pramipexole, bromocriptine	Used in combination with Levo-dopa in treatment of Parkinson's disease	• Severe cardiovascular disease • Psychotic disorders	• Nausea • Postural hypotension • Compulsive or disinhibited behaviours	Dopamine agonist, given orally
Entacapone, tolcapone	Treatment of Parkinson's disease	Phaeochromocytoma	Gastrointestinal complaints	COMT inhibitors – inhibit the peripheral breakdown of Levo-dopa by COMT enzyme

Anxiolytic agents Anxiolytic agents = substances that have a calming and therefore balancing effect on the mind, without having an antipsychotic effect.

! *Risk of psychological, but not physical dependency.*

Tab. 28 Anxiolytic agents

Active ingredient/trade names	Indications	Contraindications	Side effects	Comments
Diazepam Valium **Flunitrazepam** Rohypnol **Flurazepam** Dalmadorm **Nitrazepam** Mogadan, Imeson **Midazolam** **Triazolam** **Oxazepam** **Lorazepam**	• States of anxiety and agitation • Sleep disorders • Preparation for anaesthesia • Muscle tension • Epilepsy (clonazepam)	• Myasthenia gravis • Liver and kidney damage • Alcohol consumption • Before and during birth	• Decreased energy and difficulties concentrating • Psychological dependency • Paradoxical excitation (particularly with elderly people) • Respiratory depression at high doses • Increase in appetite • Increased risk of fall • Effect of alcohol and centrally acting drugs enhanced	• Sedative • Provides relief for anxiety and stress • Sleep-promoting • Antispasmodic • Muscle relaxant

Neuroleptic agents Neuroleptic agents = medicines with antipsychotic effect. Their main indications are **psychoses** (e.g., schizophrenia) and **states of agitation, excitability** (e.g., mania). In the following, w stands for weak (potency < 1), m for medium-strength (potency 1–5) and st for strong (potency > 10) neuroleptics.

Tab. 29 Neuroleptics

Active ingredient/ trade names	Indications	Contraindications	Side effects	Comments
Promethazine (w) Atosil **Levomepromazine** (w) Neurocil **Haloperidol** (st) Haldol	• Schizophrenia • Neuroleptanalgesia • Toxic and senile psychoses • Premedication for anaesthesia • Concomitant medication in the event of severe pain	• Glaucoma • Liver and kidney damage • Cardiovascular disease • Alcohol consumption • Parkinsonism	• Extrapyramidal and motor disorders • Malignant neuroleptic syndrome (rare) • Sedation • Anticholinergic effect • Prolactin level ↑	• Antipsychotic • Sedative • Antiemetic

Note: Page numbers followed by "*t*" indicate, tables.

Index—Active ingredients (substances)

Note: Page numbers followed by "*t*" indicate, tables.

Note: Page numbers followed by *"t"* indicate, tables.